Author's Background: Published food and wellness writer. Pescatarian recipe developer. Adult and teenage yoga teacher. Certified Reiki Level 2 practitioner and certified trauma-releasing exercises practitioner. I have written for Bahrain this Month and the Gulf Daily News, and I am now marrying my years of experience in pescatarian recipe writing, yoga teaching, and somatic shaking into one transformational wellness book.

Education:

September 2015
Masters of Science in Middle East Politics – Merit School of Oriental and African Studies, University of London
London, United Kingdom

May 2010
Bachelor of Arts in Economics
University of Victoria – Second Class
Victoria, British Columbia, Canada

May 2019
Certified RYT 200 Yoga Teacher by Yoga Alliance USA One year experience teaching yoga at Pure Yoga & Cycle (2020).

One Year experience teaching somatic yoga and trauma-releasing shaking (2020).

September 2015
Nutrition for everyday living certification The College of Naturopathic Medicine London, UK

September 2015
Cuisine Techniques Certification Le Cordon Bleu London, UK

One year experience writing pescetarian recipes for Bahrain This Month (2020).

May 2019
Frank Arjava Institute Japanese Reiki Level 2 Certified Practitioner

To the therapists I worked with and interviewed, who made my healing and this book possible. Thank you for your collaboration in helping spread mental health awareness across the GCC region.

To my publishing team. Thank you for seeing me through the production process and believing in my ideas.

Razan Ali

TRANSFORMATIVE WELLNESS

Soul Retrievals, Somatic Yoga,
Trauma Releasing Exercises,
and Ayahuasca

AUSTIN MACAULEY PUBLISHERS™
LONDON • CAMBRIDGE • NEW YORK • SHARJAH

Copyright © Razan Ali 2024

The right of Razan Ali to be identified as author of this work has been asserted by the author in accordance with Federal Law No. (7) of UAE, Year 2002, Concerning Copyrights and Neighboring Rights.

All rights reserved. No part of this publication may be reproduced, stored in a retrieval system, or transmitted in any form or by any means, electronic, mechanical, photocopying, recording, or otherwise, without the prior permission of the publishers.

Any person who commits any unauthorized act in relation to this publication may be liable to legal prosecution and civil claims for damages.

The age group that matches the content of the books has been classified according to the age classification system issued by the Ministry of Culture and Youth.

ISBN - 9789948777618 - (Paperback)
ISBN - 9789948777625 - (E-Book)

Application Number: MC-10-01-9623118
Age Classification: E

First Published 2024
AUSTIN MACAULEY PUBLISHERS FZE
Sharjah Publishing City
P.O Box [519201]
Sharjah, UAE
www.austinmacauley.ae
+971 655 95 202

To my archangels, who guide my life journey, my healing, and my work. Thank you for bringing this sage wisdom out into the world.

Publication Proposal

1. Shamanic soul retrievals, ayahausca, the Soul movement method, and TRE/EMDR therapies are newly innovative in the GCC region. Most of the therapists I worked with are located in London/US. I couldn't find their services in Bahrain or Dubai. The book's collaborating therapists are inexpensive, accessible, and performable at-home exercises (TRE/Somatic yoga), through zoom sessions (Soul retrievals/Soul movement) that clients in the GCC can seek through direct bookings with the therapist's website.
2. The primary goal of this book is to educate GCC populations between the ages of 15–40 about new transformational therapies from US/London writers, practitioners, and inventors that are unpopular or unheard of in our region. The secondary goal of this book is to encourage self-healing, self-help, and self-empowerment through Zoom therapy sessions and at-home exercises. To bring mental health awareness to the forefront of self-care in the GCC and complementary to the pre-existing prioritization of diet and exercise.

3. Target audiences are lifestyle magazines and mental health magazines in Dubai/Abu Dhabi/Bahrain. Reiki and yoga students and clients in Dubai/Bahrain. Psychotherapy goers who are interested in self-improvement and learning innovative new therapies for positive self-transformation. Target audience between the ages of 15–40.
4. Why are the book therapies innovative, not classical, and how can they be applied to the target audience? Yoga students can add somatics to their classic Hatha/Vinyasa routines at home. Traditional yoga does not target the nervous system meanwhile TRE/Somatic yoga directly affects stress/fight or flight/anxiety and can immensely calm a student and release emotional baggage. Reiki spa clients and crystal goers can explore shamanic soul retrievals, a much more powerful form of energy healing. Aromatherapy and herbal vitamin goers can venture into ayahausca (Brazilian Amazon Mushrooms), that have a healing effect on the nervous system, improve mental focus, and support cathartic emotional healing. Psychotherapy goers can add TRE/EMDR brain and body work to their traditional talk therapy to help process stuck traumatic memories in the amygdala and stuck traumatic freeze/fight or flight responses in their tight bodies and nervous systems.
5. How will I track book statistics? Coming from an economic background, I probably create Excel figures and graphs to track book publisher' sold copies over the period of years/months. If published or featured in a lifestyle magazine, sold copies

(numbers) can be tracked to correlate with indicate interest. Social media analytics on Instagram, Twitter, and LinkedIn business accounts can also be used to track gender, age group, and location. Google searches can show mentions of the author and the book on social media and in magazines.

6. To market the book, I would use Dubai media city contacts, at Al Arabiya, for example, if I score a day job there because I'm an economic/political reporter by day. I would also use the Gulf Daily News in Bahrain and Bahrain this Month (magazines, and newspapers I've written for) to market the book. I would also use Live Healthy magazine in Abu Dhabi; a feature with them would target my mental health audience. Advertise with Reiki healers I worked with in Dubai and Bahrain. Advertise with Soul Yoga and Cycle, whom I've taught yoga with in Bahrain. Advertise with the insights therapy clinic in Bahrain Financial Harbor, whom I've worked with. Advertise with Frans Pagnier in Brazil and Hawaii, with Tal Shai in California, and with Sara Haworth in London.

7. Why is this book unique from other books in the GCC region and around the world? There are plenty of Reiki, yoga, and pescatarian books published across the world in the range on 7–15 books in each topic. There are only two somatics books published by Jordan Dann: Somatic Therapy for Healing Trauma, and by Manuela Mischke-Reeds: Somatic Psychotherapy Toolbox. Only David Berceli writes about trauma-releasing exercises because he invented them in his two books, Trauma-Releasing Exercises

and Shake It Off, and in his military training exercises across the world. Sandra Ingerman is the only valid authority on shamanic soul retrievals; she published one book, Soul Retrieval: Mending the Fragmented Self, and she runs practitioner training programs across the world. The soul movement method was invented by Tal Shai, and she hasn't written a book about it yet, so it's being introduced for the first time in a book by the therapist herself, through my interview. Not to mention that the above-mentioned inventors, writers, and practitioners are not located in the GCC. So this is the first book targeting the aforementioned topics by a GCC author for a GCC audience.

Chapter One
Somatic Yoga

Somatic yoga is traditional Hatha, Vinyasa, Power, Yin yoga flows, and hypno-trance breathing, but catered toward your nervous system. Great for anxiety, increasing blood flow, opening your hips, promoting flexibility, increasing heart rate, opening your shoulders, strengthening your biceps, easing indigestion, soothing back aches, and grounding you into the present. The fastest way to relax in a mere 30 to 60 minutes is with a quick yoga flow. I've combined my years of teaching experience, therapy, and yoga certifications into two customized yoga flows that are safe and suitable for home workouts. The two flows are not recommended for pregnant women or patients with high blood pressure; please follow prenatal yoga therapists for customized instructions. Patients with orthopedic surgeries can perform yoga poses, but according to their range of motion. I would recommend steering clear of exercises one month post-surgery, taking up gentle yoga three months post-surgery, and doing Hatha/Vinyasa classes normally six months post-surgery. If you have range and mobility issues (for example, shoulder mobility like I had after orthopedic surgery), you can perform yoga poses but limit your range of motion (for example, triangle pose with your arms less straight or a block under your shoulder blades in fish pose). If you hold emotional trauma in your body (even without surgery), you'll likely have tight hips and shoulders. You can use blocks in pigeon pose under your sitting bones, for example, if your hips aren't open enough to reach the floor. Other adjustments include blocks under your crotch muscles to support a split if you can't reach the floor. A yoga ball for wheels if you can't do without. Your flexibility will come back with trauma-releasing exercises and yoga practice, but it'll take a year of consistent weekly classes. The latter flows are perfectly suited to teenagers aged 15 and above, along with adults (aged 20 to 50, who are heart healthy), and are looking for increased flexibility, back ache release, cardio, and anxiety relief. All you need is a sweat-resistant yoga mat, a yoga ball, a foam roller, and some supportive blocks (especially if inflexible) to practice these flows at home. Listen to your body and stop if you feel pain, needle sensations, or numbness at any point in your practice. The somatic flow is an express flow catered toward advanced flexibility with poses like wheel, front splits, and beginner-friendly headstands. The somatic flow includes warm-ups like Psoas releases and Trauma-releasing exercises and is excellent at easing anxiety quickly.

Advanced flexibility Somatic Flow (30 minutes):

1. Psoas release (a muscle that stretches between your abs, hips, and groin holding most of your anxiety and inflexibility). Sit in a butterfly, lifting your legs up against a wall (in butterfly) while your back rests on the floor. Stay in this position for 5 minutes to open your glutes.

2. Get into somatic cat and cow. On all fours, start moving your neck in slow circles, then move your hips in circles until you feel hip tightness from the psoas release dissipate.
3. TRE Shaking: Start trauma-releasing exercises by lying on your back and slowly pulling your legs up from the floor while in a reclining bound angle pose until you feel yourself shaking. Your ankles can rest on the floor in a butterfly while your body shakes (abs, legs, chest). To decrease the intensity of shaking, place the soles of your feet on the floor mid-shaking, and the shaking will move from your abs, chest, hips, and abs to your legs solely. Both ankles on the floor and feet on the floor shaking will release trauma from your vagus nerve, which is responsible for regulating your central nervous system and controlling the functions of your heart, digestion, and reproductive organs. Shake in 2-minute segments nonstop, then rest in butterfly or Savasana (corpse pose). Repeat the 2-minute segments four times; a total of 8 minutes should be enough (less is more with shaking because it's taxing). The softer your shakes, the less trauma you hold in your body and the better your flexibility. The more aggressive your shakes, the more trauma and tightness you hold in your chest and hips. Over time (six months to a year), and with continuous once-a-week shaking practice, you should go from aggressive shakes to soft shakes, and you should hit fitness and flexibility goals like a full split.
4. Standing flow: Sumo squat with your arms between your legs stretched backwards toward your ankles

(repeat five times, and make sure your knees are at a 90-degree comfortable angle). While standing, get into chair pose (like sitting on a chair, feet slightly apart, knees at a 90-degree angle). Start rolling your elbows with mild pressure up and down your hips while breathing in and out through your mouth. Relax and bring your heart rate down in a forward-facing wide-legged pose: legs widespread while standing, lower your upper body head to the floor, relax your arms to the floor, and let loose. Start swinging your arms left and right with your fingers intertwined.

5. 90/90, Pigeon, pelvic yoga ball, Wheel pose: Get into 90/90 pose while sitting with your spine straight to open your hips. Do 90/90 once on each side. Then get into pigeon (start on all fours, lift your left leg upwards to stretch, then bring your left leg forward to sit your left hip in 90 degrees, extend and straighten your right leg backward (on the floor), and relax sitting (spine straight) or sleeping (upper body forward, head to mat). Repeat the pigeon pose once on each side. Grab your inflated yoga ball and sit on it with your legs widespread, spine straight, and knees comfortable at 90 degrees to avoid injuries. Start jumping your pelvis up and down the ball, feeling the sinking pressure after 20 jumps. Stop the jumping and start forming pelvic circles to the right 10 times and to the left 10 times. Get into wheel by getting into goddess squat pose and balancing your back against the yoga ball. Start moving your back upwards, rolling yourself backward against the yoga ball until your hands reach the floor behind you (head upside

down between your shoulders), shoulders are externally rotated in full wheel. Balance your open hips, feet firmly on the floor, hands on the floor, shoulders externally rotated, head upside down, and chest fully open until the blood rushes to your head and you feel lightheaded.

6. Sit on a foam roller, sitting muscles comfortable, and cross your right leg on your straightened left leg. Start rolling your hips back and forth, feeling the hip tightness ease.

7. Front splits: Place your left leg on your foam roller and extend your left leg straight in front of you. Move your right leg into 90/90 (outward hip rotation, knee slightly bent). From there, start straightening your right leg fully (while maintaining outward hip/knee flexion). Stop when you feel you'll pull your hamstrings (front thigh muscles). Practice makes perfect with splits. The more you shake, the more flexible your split becomes, and warm-ups make a difference in your flexibility, so follow the somatic flow. Be patient with your splits; it takes one year of shaking and splitting to achieve them.

8. Beginner friendly headstands/handstands: Finish your workout with a Pilates handstand. Climb your feet on the wall while your hands are balanced firmly on the floor. Start with a beginner-friendly wall plank and move your hands closer to the wall and your legs further up the wall as you go into a more advanced handstand. To come out of your handstand, simply move your hands forward away from the wall and legs slowly down the wall and jump down. For a

beginner-friendly headstand, try balancing on your bed; it's softer and safer for your neck. Get into a forearm plank and balance your head between your interlocked fingers while in a forearm plank. Move your legs up your bed's headboard with your hips in a frog position (less pressure on your neck than legs straight). To come out of your headstand, bring your frog knees down to the bed, then release your headlock plank.

Chapter Two

Energy healing (soul retrievals, body codes, and soul movements)
Haworth, Sara (2022) *Quoted Interview with Sara Haworth (London Soul Retrieval Shaman).*
www.sara-haworth.com

    I have been practicing core shamanism since 2001 and traditional Mexihka healing since 2004. I came to training as a healer starting in 1997, when I was looking for ways to help myself beyond the psychotherapies that were on offer at the time. I wanted something that was more integrated with the body and soul, and I felt that earth-based spirituality had great healing potential. For me, it is an ongoing process; we never stop learning, and it is important for me to approach the work with a 'beginners' mind.'

    In order to be of help to one's community, I believe it is best to have a thorough grounding in the practices, a sense of lineage, and the support of peers who can be counted on for support and challenge in an appropriate measure. This is more important than years of training, although insight is also built by experience. But sometimes the most beautiful healing can be received from someone recently trained who is coming from their heart and is not clouded by status or reputation.

My own work in the Mexican tradition follows my teacher, Miahuatzin Buendia Sanchez, who is from the DF area, close to Teotihuacan. She has an apprenticeship that consists of 13 seminars and is a comprehensive process of learning through oral teaching, physical practice, and ceremony such as temascal (sweat lodge). Her emphasis is on service and self-knowledge in order to best use one's abilities for the people who come for healing.

As a European, I don't have any direct contact with tribes or with sourcing plants, including medicine plants. I am mindful of the need for protection for people's land, the plants themselves, which have been over-exploited in recent times, and for the survival of tribal customs, traditions, and languages. There is a tension between wanting to widen inclusion and create access to traditional healing and avoiding exploitation and cultural appropriation. My own meeting with Miahuatzin was first in London, as she undertook to come to Europe, supported in her decision by her own teachers and community. Although I have been to Mexico many times, I am only ever a visitor, and I respect the direction of my teacher and her community in interacting with people, plants, and traditional ceremonies.

First, we have to be open to the idea of a very different way of perceiving the world, which is both a brain state and a cultural shift away from what core shamanic practitioners have called 'ordinary reality.' We all have a sense of our soul, but it can be very hard to put into words. Soul retrieval is a term used to describe a ceremony in which a healer journeys (undergoes a shift of perception) to find the essence of a person that may have been lost through acute or prolonged situations of suffering, including accidents, shocks, frights, and illness, as well as emotional traumas and inherited wounds. It is a visionary practice with a focus on the power of nature to heal and guide us. In traditional earth-based cultures, humans are not separate from the earth and from other species. Inter-species communication is possible, including with animals, plants, trees, and the elements. The contemporary shamanic practitioner or healer seeks to reconnect the person with an innate self and with the earth while honoring the complexity of psychology and cultural identity. There is no one way to be human, but we can recognize when we feel well and whole.

In the conventions of shamanic healing, there are three worlds: the middle, the lower, and the upper. These have been widely written about, so I won't repeat anything here, only to say that often it is the lower world that we visit for soul retrieval, and we find wisdom, sacred knowledge, and guidance from teachers in the upper world. In my experience, there are many dimensions to be visited, but the process of naming or mapping them would be difficult because cosmological visions are specific to peoples and places; we are oriented by our environment and can access our own guides and symbols.

Personally, because of the diversity and range of clients, I like to have a good conversation with someone coming to see me in order to get background information. It is a kind of preparation for the ceremony itself, and the most important aspect of the conversation is gaining permission to work in areas of pain and vulnerability, as well as building trust and preparing for the return of vital energy. It is possible to perceive someone's suffering, but they may not be ready to focus on it or receive the healing in that moment. I think this may be a difference from more traditional healers, who are working with a community of kinship and belonging – they will have a shared language and common experience and may be able to go directly into the ceremony, connecting with spirits and healing without much need for talking.

Ancestral healing – again, it depends both on the client and the moment in which they are coming for help. The wise ones say that when we heal, we are working with seven generations past and seven generations into the future. In my experience, because of the radical changes in our world over the last 150 years or so, most of the immediate need for healing lies in these generations. Sometimes I seek an ancestor (of the client) who has not experienced trauma to be the guide for the work, and more recently, I may invite someone from the future generations who can bring reassurance to the present.

Soul retrievals can have the effect of unlocking frozen feelings, and it is important that there is enough attention given to the integration process so that the person is not left to go on a roller coaster of unexpected emotions without preparation and support. In other situations, perhaps if the person has done a lot of therapy or other kinds of healing, the effect would be less one of unfamiliar emotions and more of a reclamation of power, motivation, and dynamism. It can also be that a person is in a state of vulnerability or may be facing life circumstances and responsibilities that mean it's not the right moment for a cathartic experience. It is something that has to be discerned on the day. Having said all that, spirit guides the work, and there is no way to be completely certain of all the effects of a soul retrieval. Some of them are long-term and subtle, so that we can only see them long after the cathartic wave has passed.

I can't really talk too much about Reiki – in my experience, it transmits a deeply beautiful, warming, and relaxing energy, inviting a rebalancing and restoration of harmony. But I am not a Reiki master or teacher – I was initiated by Torsten Lange, and I do recommend looking at his work; he has a lot to say about the depths of the possibilities of Reiki. I think a significant difference is 'story' – in shamanic healing and soul retrieval, we engage with a person's lived experience, their origins, and ancestry in terms of a story that can be retraced, mended, and made whole. In my training with Sandra Ingerman, one of the leading teachers of shamanism and soul retrieval, we were taught that the healing story was a vital part of the ceremony. Through the retrieval of energy that was lost, e.g., joy, love of music and dancing, or singing, we shift the emphasis from a story of trauma to one of recovery and thriving. It is a dynamic process; we may not tie everything up neatly, but we can reach a state in which we can contemplate our trauma or talk about it without reawakening and re-experiencing the trauma itself. There is also the integration of the shamanic ceremony, in which we honor the earth and our ancestors by giving thanks for the healing and taking other steps that have been suggested to us through the healing as a way to deepen our connection and to become empowered on our own spiritual paths.

Each soul retrieval is a very personal and distinctive experience, no two are exactly alike, even for the same client. And as I said before, you can't really predict the impact of a soul retrieval in too much detail because it really is a spiritual process. However, in the short term, people can experience lightness, joy, even elation, or a feeling of calm, groundedness, presence in their bodies, and a greater ability to feel, to have a sense of autonomy and solidity that may have been missing before. Following the ceremony, they can have serendipitous experiences, clarity, a feeling of connection, and 'rightness.' They may notice things in nature that seem relevant, have powerful dreams, or have happy coincidences as things realign. I always ask for feedback a while after the session so that people have a chance to check back in and share what has been changing for them. Many people report increased confidence and a sense of direction; they may have changed homes, jobs, or resolved relationship issues. With family members, they may have better boundaries, improved relationships, or have greater support. I often work with people who want to unlock their creativity or complete projects and dreams that have been blocked, including having children, completing a qualification, or changing careers. So often it is fear, a feeling of lack, or self-doubt that has been generated by unresolved trauma, and when we do this kind of healing, we don't forget the hurt, but we are no longer governed by it. We can choose. One of the most rewarding things that people report is finding their own spiritual path, deepening their own connection to whatever guides them, and a greater sense of trust in their own abilities.

Clients reach me from all over the world – that is perhaps one of the few blessings that has come out of the pandemic, that we are now more connected globally via the internet. I have worked with people in the US, throughout Europe, the UAE, Egypt, and, of course, Bahrain! My clients are all kinds of people, but I think the common factor is that they are willing to be open to new experiences and they want to grow emotionally and spiritually.

Chapter Three

The Brazilian Amazon (Ayahausca, dragon's blood, Echinacea)
Pagnier, Frans (2022) *Paraphrased Interview with Frans Pagnier, Owner of Sacred Snuff shops in Brazil and Hawaii.* Sacred-Snuff.com

Frans Pagnier Introduction: Sacred Connections Founder Frans Pagnier owns two shops in Brazil and Hawaii. A Netherlands Native who has lived in Brazil for ten years, he was introduced to the Yawanawa tribe chief while visiting the Brazilian Amazon Mountains. It is through his friendship with tribal chiefs that his snuff collection was hand-picked and supplied to his sacred connection shops. The Hawaii shop started as a collaboration with a friend of Frans from the States. Both shops now supply to the US market, the Eastern European market, Africa, and the Middle East. Sacred snuff is popular among psychotherapists, who integrate its cathartic healing qualities into their sessions. World-class Hawaiian surfers use snuff to help them concentrate. Business and corporate leaders are also customers, so their client base is varied.

The Sacred Connections shop supplies different types of snuff called rape (pronounced hape). Some blends are more grounding and strong, others more feminine and gentle. Some blends heal colds, boost immunity, and anti-ageing while other blends clear energy centers, clear the evil eye, and clear negativity in your energy field. Some blends are great for depression, and other blends are great for anxiety. Some are for women's reproductive health, while others can calm down anxious children. So it depends on your needs what snuff you should order, but all snuffs open energy centers, open pineal glands, and hit nervous system glands in your nose, throat, and brain, which explains the meditative and sometimes deep cathartic experience that can come from taking them. Snuff is administered with a bamboo pipe (kuripe) by blowing with your mouth through one end and into your nose with the other end. Administer a pea-sized amount in each nostril (take a 10-minute break between nostrils) and breathe through your mouth while letting your nose and throat release phlegm. If you need tissues for your phlegm or need to vomit, do so; it's a normal part of the physical cleanse ritual. If you took a starter pea-sized amount in each nostril, the snuff should cause relaxation, concentration, and meditation. If you took a larger amount (two pea sizes each nostril), then expect to go into a panic attack or depressive episode lasting 15 minutes before it wears off, and you are left with a tobacco high lasting two hours. Larger amounts of snuff are recommended for more advanced users who have the therapy tools to navigate through cathartic feelings. I personally took a larger amount at first and used my association tools, trauma-releasing exercises, heart-opening poses like the wheel, and Reiki energy healing to help move the cathartic panic and sadness through my body. When I calmed down after 15 minutes, I did the second nostril. Start with the right nostril (death) and finish with the left nostril (rebirth). Take a 15-minute break between nostrils to process your emotions, and use the therapy tools mentioned above. After 30 minutes and after processing the phlegm, vomit, panic, and sadness coming up from both nostrils and my nervous system, I used association exercises and my Echinacea tincture to calm myself down. Trauma-releasing exercises are discussed in Chapter six, so have a read there for the interview with my psychotherapist, who's certified in TRE and EMDR. The reason Jagube snuff creates panic and sadness when taken in large doses is because the ayahausca plant hits your central nervous system. It hits your vagus nerve, which controls your digestion, heart, and reproductive organs. So if you feel a vibration in your heart or crying, it's a normal heart healing. If you feel energy in your uterus or hips or need to go into splits to stretch, it's a normal pelvic healing. If you vomit, it's a normal digestion response. Sometimes we hold anger in our stomachs, but we also hold unhealthy friend foods, and Jagube's energy is cleansing and detoxing one. On the bright side of the unpleasant cathartic purge is a more flexible body, vegetarian healthy cravings, and a more open heart emotionally (less defensive and more forgiving toward yourself and others). Emotional trauma can make us defensive, able to relate sexually but not emotionally to our partners, and that is how trauma bonds based on emotional unavailability, insensitivity, lying, and cheating are created. Echinacea is a flower used as a muscle relaxant for your hips and shoulders; it's also a stress and inflammation acidity reducer, and is being studied for its anti-cancer properties. I use my Echinacea tincture from flower essences at Iherb to calm myself down every morning with water. It's a good idea to take an Echinacea tincture (two spritzes in warm jasmine tea) after your Jagube panic attack episode because it will calm and stabilize you. Another exercise you can try to calm down and stabilize is association. Looking around the room, slowly turning your neck. Look at the ceiling, floor, and walls slowly, noticing the details. When you are in the now, you cannot be anxious, and when you can see, smell, or sense your surroundings, you feel safe.

Jagube is made from the Ayahausca vine (inhibitors) and mixed with tobacco, so it has harmaline but no psychedelic DMT. It's legal and safe to use at home, and the trip lasts 5–15 minutes depending on the dosage. Ayahausca tea is made from the bark (alkaloids), not mixed with tobacco, and contains the psychedelic DMT, so you might start seeing colors and feel deeply cathartic purging, but DMT is unsafe to use at home and is illegal to import. An Ayahausca tea trip lasts four hours with more intense visions and deeper healing (panic and crying episodes). Ayahausca bark tea is only legal in Brazil under the supervision of a tribal shaman, and so indulging in it is costly and inconveniently long distance. Meanwhile, Jagube snuff is legal to import, mild, safe, and much less expensive and traumatic, while still able to induce deep cathartic releases the way trauma-releasing exercises, EMDR, or energy healing sessions do. The concept of heal it to feel it is prominent in psychotherapy and energy healing, meaning you have to feel the panic attacks and sadness stuck in your nervous system to release, and heal. You have to regulate your nervous system from high alert (trauma response), otherwise known as anxiety (fight), or depression (flight). Our natural nervous system can switch between relaxed and alert, but when we've experienced child abuse, we can get stuck in high alert 24/7, which is high stress and high inflammation, creating physical and mental health problems like arthritis, gastritis, uterus abnormalities, hormonal irregularities, palpitations, and even surgeries. Our vagus nerve governs our organs and systems, and so a dysregulated vagus nerve will create physical problems in our physical organs. The goal is to retrain our nervous system to go from alert back to relaxed. You can do this with somatic yoga, a challenging yoga pose followed by a relaxing yoga pose; you can do this with ayahausca, a cathartic release followed by a self-soothing meditative state; you can do this with TRE, a nervous system relaxed high followed by an anger episode; and you can do it through EMDR, a panic attack childhood memory followed by tracing a light that reprocesses memories and calms you down. The goal is to go back to a relaxed nervous system as nature intended, as opposed to being stuck in high alert the way trauma intended.

There are different tribes and different snuff producers on the sacred connections website (sacred-snuff.com). Snuff producers don't have to isolate or follow special diets to produce the tobacco dried vine, but they need knowledge of shamanic traditions, knowledge of the Amazon forest, and knowledge of the plants to be able to hand make snuff. The most popular snuffs on the sacred snuff website are Forca feminina from the Yawanawa tribe; the producer is the tribal chief's daughter, and her snuff carries a feminine, gentle quality. Yawanawa tribe's New Hope is produced by a tribe member now living in the city who has fled to escape tribal alcoholism and community diseases. Kutanawa tribe Heart of the Boa snuff is another best seller. Made from the Sapota tree, which has heart-shaped leaves, it protects from negativity, jealousy, and spiritual attacks. Lastly, my favorite snuff, Jagube, from the Ayahausca tree, is famed for its central nervous system healing qualities, excellent for processing panic and depression, great for mediation and focus, and can help retrain your nervous system by releasing traumatic stuck emotions.

Store the snuff in a dry, dark place away from humidity and heat. Snuff keeps well in desert climates for up to a year, but keeps only 3–6 months in humid climates like Brazilian rain forests. I recommend getting through your snuff within three months of opening it because it starts to rot. So, for example, a 10 ml bottle used consistently once a week for three months should use up the bottle before it rots. Lastly, dragon's blood is an antimicrobial liquid that drips out of its tree bark in the Brazilian Amazon. It's red in color, similar to a tonic, and has blood-cleansing qualities as well as regenerative qualities for both your internal organs and external cuts. It helps stop bleeding; it's used to clean wounds; and it can clot the skin in only 20 minutes.

Recommended snuffs to buy on sacred-snuff.com (they ship through UPS internationally, and it takes two weeks.)

Yawanawa – Forca feminina

Yawanawa – New Hope

Kuntanawa – Heart of the Boa

Puyanawa – Jagube

Chapter Four

Psychotherapy (trauma-releasing exercises and EMDR for PTSD)

Nervous system regulation is of utmost importance in body trauma healing, and trauma-releasing exercises are great at regulating the nervous system, regulating emotional healing, and bringing flexibility back into the body. I learned about TRE when I visited a psychologist with the intention of regulating my nervous system after childhood abuse, molestation, and beatings. TRE, created by Dr. David Berceli, is a natural muscle reflex that both humans and animals have, which shakes trauma out of the nervous system with the intention of healing it. Shaking tremors, which start from the Bakasana yoga pose, lift your knees slowly off the floor till your body starts shaking automatically. These tremors can be mild or strong, and you can control their intensity through the placement of your ankles. Ankles placed sideways on the floor will result in stronger tremors, and feet placed flat on the floor (ankles straight) will result in softer tremors. When you first start shaking, you'll notice stronger tremors because you hold more trauma in your body, and a stronger emotional release in the form of anger, crying, or panic will follow. This is normal because an emotional release is healing and will eventually lead you to a place of peace and joy. As you practice shaking once a week for six months, you'll notice a change in your body's flexibility. If you were stiff before you started, you'll feel your hips open, and you'll perform yoga splits with ease. You'll eventually feel more confident and less isolated with no emotional reaction after shaking because you've felt your anger/sadness/panic consistently and released it. Your emotional trauma triggers, in a sense, will be processed, healed, and released. The immediate (15-minute) after effects of shaking also include relaxation and the reduction of anxiety.

David Berceli's website describes his TRE technique as follows:

'TRE® is an innovative series of exercises that assist the body in releasing deep muscular patterns of stress, tension, and trauma. The exercises safely activate a natural reflex mechanism of shaking or vibrating that releases muscular tension, calming down the nervous system. When this muscular shaking/vibrating mechanism is activated in a safe and controlled environment, the body is encouraged to return to a state of balance.'

'Tension and Trauma Releasing Exercises (or TRE®) are based on the fundamental idea, backed by research, that stress, tension, and trauma are both psychological and physical. TRE®'s reflexive muscle vibrations generally feel pleasant and soothing. After doing TRE®, many people report feelings of peace and well-being. TRE® has helped many thousands of people globally.' Berceli, David (May 3, 2005). *Trauma-Releasing Exercises*. Book Surge Publishing.

Traumaprevention.com

My experience with TRE was as follows: I went in inflexible, with tight hips that couldn't yoga split and unprocessed childhood emotions like anxiety, depression, and anger. When I first started shaking, my shakes were violent, and followed after one week with an emotional release. As I progressed to the six-month mark, I noticed a difference in my body and feelings. I would no longer feel anger, crying, or panic after shaking, and my shakes became soft and less violent, and I was flexible enough to do my yoga splits. So shaking will release your emotional trauma (from sexual/physical abuse or surgical trauma) if practiced weekly in the span of six to eight months. Just feel your feelings when they come up, and don't suppress with alcohol, food, or sex while practicing your tremors consistently (once a week). I do my shaking before my yoga weekly to open up my body before splits.

EMDR is a light therapy targeted toward your amygdala (emotional brain), where childhood trauma is still stored and unprocessed. Eye movement desensitization and reprocessing is a psychotherapy tool used to process traumatic and painful memories that cause post-traumatic stress disorder. EMDR aims to reduce symptoms of trauma by changing how your memories are stored in your brain. An EMDR therapist does this by leading you through a series of side-to-side eye movements as you recall traumatic memories in small segments until those memories no longer cause a reaction. For me, EMDR triggered childhood panic and sadness associated with painful childhood molestation and beatings. After my panic attack or depression episode, the EMDR light would soothe me into a state of relaxation. So the light not only brings up the painful memory for you to feel it, but it also reprocesses the memory, allowing you to feel soothed. I did a total of 12 TRE and EMDR sessions with my therapist and continued to practice TRE weekly at home for a year, seeing flexibility results, achieving the splits after six months, and noticing an increase in confidence, happiness, and emotional stability after six months to one year.

TRE and Military PTSD:

This journal highlights the use of trauma-releasing exercises (TRE) for inducing the body's innate tremor mechanism in an Australian former soldier who experienced post-traumatic stress disorder (PTSD) after a major motor vehicle accident (MVA) in 2009. Improvements in physical and emotional wellbeing following six months of TRE is clinically significant, as was the improvement in perceived stress at four months with ongoing use of TRE. Using current evidence-based treatments, only one third of people with post-traumatic stress disorder (PTSD) recover fully, while 30–40% gain no benefit (1). Heath, R. Beattle, J. (2022). Case report of a former soldier using TRE (Tension/Trauma Releasing exercises). Journal of Military and Veterans' Health, 27(3).

https://jmvh.org/article/case-report-of-a-former-soldier-using-tre-tension-trauma-releasing-exercises-for-posttraumatic-stress-disorder-self-care/

TRE draws on The Polyvagal Theory of the nervous system. Reflexive response to threat passes through three stages from social engagement (ventral vagal), mobilization (sympathetic fight-flight), and freeze (dorsal vagal response/shutdown). Using TRE, a similarly reflexive process, but in reverse order, is thought to occur, whereby the release of the dorsal vagal freeze response results in movement (tremor/shakes) as part of the body's innate mechanism to release fight, or flight, and down-regulate to social ventral vagal. Heath, R. Beattle, J. (2022). Case report of a former soldier using TRE (Tension/Trauma Releasing exercises). *Journal of Military and Veteran' Health,* 27(3).

https://jmvh.org/article/case-report-of-a-former-soldier-using-tre-tension-trauma-releasing-exercises-for-posttraumatic-stress-disorder-self-care/

With training provided to military services in the US, Brazil, Switzerland, Norway, Austria, Ukraine, Canada, and Poland, TRE is well accepted by military personnel as a PTSD trauma healing practice that does not require a therapist once correctly taught. Heath, R. Beattle, J. (2022). Case report of a former soldier using TRE (Tension/Trauma Releasing exercises). *Journal of Military and Veterans' Health.* 27(3).

https://jmvh.org/article/case-report-of-a-former-soldier-using-tre-tension-trauma-releasing-exercises-for-posttraumatic-stress-disorder-self-care/

Chapter Five

The Soul Movement Method®
Quoted Interview with Tal Shai, Founder of The Soul Movement Method® soulmovements.com

What is the Soul Movement Method®?

The Soul Movement Method® began to solidify as a unique process in its own right during my 30 years of teaching and supervising students in a five-year-long certification program for Body-Centered and Transpersonal Psychotherapy. At that time, I was also working online as an Intuitive Business Coach, seeing clients in my private psychotherapy practice, leading peace-building and conflict resolution immersions, and developing and teaching a variety of personal development workshops. Although I was not aware of it at the time, my involvement in seemingly separate professional arenas, in addition to my background as an energy-medicine practitioner, greatly informed my evolving body-of-work.

A memorable turning point transpired when I was asked to teach a course in Advanced Transpersonal Psychology to fifth-year students of body-centered and transpersonal psychology. I was inspired to create a course that weaved the principles of Jungian psychology, integral psychology, Gestalt therapy and systems theory into the experiential framework of what was organically evolving into The Soul Movement Method®.

On completion of this advanced coursework, many of my students requested that I create a continuation course to teach them "my methodology. This was the first time I took it upon myself to outline a clearly delineated, step-by-step process of the body-of-work that had evolved through me over the years. Shortly thereafter, I began offering this process to the general public as a unique, stand-alone method. A few years later, in 2014, I finally made it official by registering it as The Soul Movement Method®.

How was my experience with the Soul Movement Method®?

I personally found that 1–2 sessions working with The Soul Movement Method® produced dramatic results around long-standing issues I was experiencing in my stomach, uterus, leg, and hip areas. As a result of our work together, I also regained my lost creativity, experienced renewed energy, and released unprocessed crying, fear, confusion, self-hate, and headaches. Within 2–6 sessions, over a period of three months, I experienced more dramatic results as compared to one year of treatment with TRE/EMDR. I started painting and sketching for the first time in my life. Moved to Dubai, a more geographically supportive environment, and wrote a five chapter wellness book I've been slacking on for four years, which details my experiences with soul retrievals, The Soul Movement Method®, EMDR/TRE, somatic yoga, and ayahausca. I moved out of my comfort zone in Bahrain and started taking action on my goals to manifest them into reality.

I got over my procrastination and fear, and my disassociated womb creativity from childhood sexual abuse quickly returned. It was surprising to see myself effortlessly write and paint while I've been blocked all my life.

How does the Soul Movement Method® work, and why is it effective so quickly?

The reason results can feel so "quick" or "surprising" or even "miraculous," is because most of us are conditioned to view issue-resolution, and life in general through a three-dimensional lens, as such expecting outcomes to follow a linear, logical, step-by-step sequence.

The Soul Movement Method®, however, is sourced in a quantum paradigm that is guided by a completely different set of principles. It is designed to help us tap into an expanded field of awareness that houses within it the entire memory bank of our personal and soul experiences to date. I have come to refer to this field as our "soul fieldTM."

Our soul fieldTM does not follow a linear or logical pattern or sequence and is organized more like a "soup of energetic impressions" that essentially fuels our emotional, mental, and physical well-being, or lack thereof. Essentially, if a soul memory were added to this soup of energetic impressions yesterday (in the past) and yet again today (in the present), both memories would exist as part of the same soup. In other words, if an ancestor seven generations back experienced unresolved trauma, that impression would have the same capacity to detract or add to our well-being as would a childhood memory or wound. Both energetic impressions, although sourced in different timelines on our soul trajectory, are experienced by our energetic body as a "lived reality."

The Soul Movement Method® harnesses the wisdom of our body, in combination with a range of proprietary tools, to "google" this soup of energetic impressions (aka our 'soul fieldTM') for specific memories associated with our unique issue, challenge, or enquiry, in service to resolving them for the very last time.

Imagine for a moment that you displaced the engine to your car and then spent years looking for it to no avail. Then, one day, you discovered a technology that was able to pinpoint its exact whereabouts. Guess what would happen once you reinstalled this engine in your car? Your car would be up and running in no time...and you would be able to drive places again. What may seem sudden or miraculous to our three-dimensional brain is actually a function of specifically pinpointing what we "lost," or rather, what we dissociated from as a result of past trauma, and then effectively "reinstalling" this part in our energetic system. Once we retrieve the part needed to affect the outcome we seek, results are immediate.

In this sense, The Soul Movement MethodTM can be likened to the soul retrieval process in Shamanic work. Once an entanglement in our soul fieldTM is resolved, we are no longer disassociated from that part. We essentially become the recipients of our own expanded flow of life-force energy entering our system. This is precisely how we regain a sense of wholeness, a process that is palpably nourishing and transformative to our entire energetic system and consequently to our lives.

Can you share surprising results that your other clients have experienced?

Anecdote #1:

One of my clients, a successful coach in her own right, won a high-ticket raffle valued at $12,000 to join a lucrative business mastermind group she had yearned to attend. Her name was singularly called out at a large weekend event of over two-thousand attendees. Since this transpired two days after her Soul Movement MappingTM Session, wherein she released a long-standing "block-to-receiving" in her maternal lineage, she was overflowing with a palpable sense of awe when she called to share this with me. Prior to this large win, she had never won anything in her life and was well aware of how synchronous and aligned this was with "the healing she experienced" a few days earlier.

Client anecdote #2:

A few days after tending to a longstanding experience of "not feeling supported by the healthy masculine," one of my clients, in her words, literally had "$5000 fall in my (her) lap" when her father spontaneously decided to sell a piece of heavy equipment from his farm and divide the proceeds amongst his children. Since he had never gifted money to her or her siblings before, she was well aware of this "miraculous" synchronicity that transpired the same week of her Soul Movement MappingTM session. She was also in awe of how the sum of money she had received was the exact amount she needed to fund the remainder of her coaching program, which she joined with the intention of healing her money wounds.

Other outcomes clients have reported include:

Resolving a relationship with a spouse after being on the "brink of divorce."Reconnecting with an estranged parent.Gaining crystal-clear clarity and inner alignment around their soul-centered niche.Feeling more empowered and effective in making financial decisions and manifesting abundance.Enrolling clients into their high-ticket (premium level) private or group offerings from a place of alignment and ease.Manifesting their soulmate.Releasing weight and loving their body.Coming out of hiding and feeling at ease around being visible (this is often sourced in ancestral survival mechanisms and fear, which can be cleared. I know this one well!).Feeling centered and calm while presenting a workshop or presentation in front of a large audience. The results clients have experienced are truly unique to them and typically correspond with their specific intentions and life journey. When we harness a larger perspective than our smaller, limited one, the sky is truly the limit.

How is The Soul Movement Method® different from EMDR/TRE?

Soul Movement Method® has the capacity to quite effectively surface root cause issues that are difficult, if not impossible, to access through body work or talk modalities alone. Since root-cause issues are typically trauma-based, it is important to work with a skilled professional who has the know-how, experience, and presence to hold for this inner material and guide you on a path toward resolution.

It is important to tend to our energetic-emotional body because it informs and affects our physical body. Treating the physical body alone can be likened to treating the fruits of a tree rather than tending to the roots that inform and affect the fruit. Both options are valid, but one option is limited and will never provide us with the long-lasting and sustainable results we seek.

- Those interested in exploring the Soul Movement Method® can book a free 15-minute consultation with Tal Shai on her website at soulmovements.com.
- You can book her 90-Day Immersion, six-session program, for a discounted investment of $1500 (full pay) or 3x payments of $540.
- Returning clients who have completed the 90-Day Immersion can book single sessions at $350.
- Soul Movement Method® sessions are conducted online through Zoom.

Citations: APA Style

1. Haworth, Sara (2022) *Quoted Interview with Sara Haworth (London Soul Retrieval Shaman).*
www.sara-haworth.com

2. Heath, R. Beattle, J. (2022). Case report of a former soldier using TRE (Tension/Trauma Releasing exercises). *Journal of Military and Veterans' Health,* 27(3).

3. https://jmvh.org/article/case-report-of-a-former-soldier-using-tre-tension-trauma-releasing-exercises-for-posttraumatic-stress-disorder-self-care/

4. Berceli, David (May 3, 2005). *Trauma-Releasing Exercises.* BookSurge Publishing.
Traumaprevention.com

5. Pagnier, Frans (2022). *Paraphrased Interview with Frans Pagnier, Owner of Sacred Snuff shops in Brazil and Hawaii.*
Sacred-Snuff.com

6. Sullivan, Courtney. Cronkelton, Emily. (September 9, 2021). *Butterfly pose sixbenefits of this classic hip opener*. Healthline.
   Healthline.com
7. Shai, Tal. (2014). *Quoted Interview with Tal Shai(Inventor of* the Soul Movement Method®).
   www.soulmovements.com

www.ingramcontent.com/pod-product-compliance
Lightning Source LLC
Chambersburg PA
CBHW030516220526
45464CB00006B/2828